5 Coins and a Cup

Wayne Harburn

ISBN 9781805176855

Publisher: Independent Publishing Network.
Publication date: 6th May 2024
ISBN: 978-1-80517-685-5
Author: Wayne Harburn
Please direct all further book orders to
5coinsandacup@gmail.com

Checkout all the pictures from Wayne's experience at
https://www.instagram.com/5coinsandacup/

Dedication

To Utochka

Table of Contents

Introduction

Just after midnight on a Thursday, I was helped into the A & E Room at the Chelsea & Westminster Hospital by my cab driver. After consuming a simple warm ham and cheese roll that left me feeling a little off, this is the story of how that simple act turned into my own personal life-threatening shit storm. A storm that involved my stomach perforate and spill its contents all over my insides, content that was usually reserved for being evacuated out of my arsehole in the direction of a toilet bowl. The next few hours saw my own personal pain meter get recalibrated as I found myself pleading to anyone in the ER to knock me out, please due to the pain. I had seen Dexter, our friendly Netflix serial killer does it all the time to his victims and they woke up just fine. Why couldn't someone do the same to me as my stomach had become akin to a washing machine filled with rocks, broken glass and fishhooks and I felt I was reaching my limits. I had lost all sense of dignity and somewhere between pleading to anyone who would listen for the gift of unconsciousness to asking God to just to kill me, I experienced a personal low. In short, I didn't die because this is the story of how I survived and went on to survive an even scarier beast, NHS post operative care.

Chapter 1

Microwaved Ham and Cheese Rolls

It was Wednesday evening and I had just sat down to enjoy two warm ham and cheese rolls that I had made for myself in the kitchen. I was staying in shared accommodation and found myself a comfy place on the sofa so I could enjoy the latest NETFLIX offering while I ate my dinner. I admit I am not in the habit of eating slowly. I finished the first roll off in a few mouthfuls and for some reason it left me feeling a little off. This surprised me as microwaved cheese and ham rolls had almost made it to "soul food" on my personal menu. I thought nothing of it and sat back to enjoy the movie

Ford vs Ferrari, a movie starring Matt Damon, someone who I had actually met years before in the movie Syriana. I had been hired as an oil consultant due to the director and I having a mutual friend, I actually had been paid to go over the script on a wet Saturday afternoon years beforehand. I remember I had to sign a non-disclosure agreement and that the driver told me to make any corrections by writing on the script and that I was to give everything back to him including all my notes once done and tell no one what I had read. I corrected things like them selling 6 million bushels of oil to barrels of oil and how one monologue that Matt Damon's character had to say about the economic impact of oil prices and petroleum economics made absolutely no sense . Since I had crossed out so much of it already, I humbly wrote the monologue myself, stapled it into the script with an apology to the academy award winning director saying that the easiest way for me to correct what I read was just write it out as I think it made sense. I mentioned that I was not a writer and was just trying to be helpful and that they could call me if they needed to. The script also contained a few stories from people I had introduced the director to months beforehand when he was doing his research. Stories that had been told to him off the record, stories that made me wonder what the result of them being told in a movie would be as some of the goings on in the oil industry are not for public consumption.

Suddenly I was happy to be under the NDA and the term plausible deniability came to mind. The surprising unexpected highlight came when I saw the movie in Miami with my girlfriend, firstly none of the stories that I was concerned about had made it to the final cut of the movie, the fact that I can be seen for a millisecond was ok but when Matt Damon said the monologue that I had typed out that rainy Saturday afternoon in London almost 2 years beforehand, I was left gobsmacked. So that was my brush with Hollywood and now I was seeing Matt Damon play Carrol Shelby in a movie where Lee Iococa was a character that I had also once met. With all this nostalgia I was surprised that I wasn't feeling better. I actually felt awful. I was even more surprised when I decided to go upstairs to lay down as I hate starting a movie and not watching it to the end. Upstairs was also 5 flights of stairs away.

It was now about 11pm and earlier that day I had asked a friend of mine to allow me to use her bank account details as my phone was having problems making payments and I had told her I would give her the cash that evening. I also wanted to see my friend as I know giving her cash for any reason makes her smile. My mode of transport at the time was my electric skateboard (12kg) which I grabbed and then proceeded to carry down the stairs, at the same time thinking I must be more careful about my choice of ham and rolls since my stomach was definitely not settling properly.

I was hoping a late-night skate over to my friend's house would set me right. I always enjoy riding my electric skateboard around London at night and always feel it is a privilege. Anyone who has ever ridden a skateboard must agree that riding a skateboard around London's streets is something to be savoured. I started doing it during the lockdown which put so many London Cab Drivers out of work. I was forced to close my business during the lockdown and there were many tough days. The empty streets during lockdown gave me the opportunity to clock up nearly 2000 km of travel on my board. No matter how bad my day was I always thought skateboarding home through London's empty streets felt like something special and was often the highlight of my day. It still made me feel good and along with all the winks, passing smiles and thumbs up from cabbies, drivers and pedestrians indicating that they would love to be joining me, this more than outweighed the few negative comments I had received over the past few years. Comments like "You're old enough to know better", "You're crazy riding that thing at your age", and my personal favourite from a man who lived in my building who confronted me one day to tell me "You have no respect for how bad the driver who kills you will feel when he runs you over and kills you dead". "I will be dead" I thought. He obviously had a strong belief in the afterlife and the capacity for a soul to carry guilt, for me I doubt it. With that I dragged my board down the 5 flights of stairs and set off into the night.

A few minutes later I was out the front of my friend's house and was surprised that I was feeling a little faint, and my stomach was making some odd noises. I pressed the buzzer and proceeded to carry my board up the first flight of stairs. Getting to the first landing the board seemed a lot heavier than it usually was, so I left it on the landing. As I started up the second flight of stairs, I remember my friend opening her front door only to find that rather than having climbed up the flight of stairs, I was now laid out on the stairs, my legs having failed to obey my commands. She immediately helped me up to her apartment. After giving her the cash which did make her smile, she laid me on her sofa and said she was going to take care of me. She prided herself on always being prepared and kept all sorts of energy shots in her fridge for just such occasions. Seeing that I needed something strong she offered me some new energy shot followed by a Red Bull plus one other shot and strangely I was feeling better in no time. I thanked my friend and feeling my Red Bull wings, I grabbed my board, went down the stairs and headed back into the night.

Arriving back where I was staying, I climbed the 5 flights of stairs up to my room. I was once again reminded by Mr Newton that gravity sucks. Once in my room I put my board on charge, it was now official. I truly felt like shit. The energy drink high had gone, my stomach was making all sorts of sounds and after moaning to my roommate, I mentioned to him that I felt terrible and that I was going to go to the chemist. He agreed I looked terrible and told me to take it easy. As I staggered down the 5 flights of stairs, I found it strange how much I was sweating, "I really do need to work out more" I thought to myself. I finally flagged a cab and then I realized it was after midnight and given the only place I could think of getting relief was the Accident and Emergency centre at the Chelsea and Westminster hospital, The A&E at the C&W was my chosen destination We got there and damn it, I had forgotten my phone, I asked the driver how much was the fare and as he hurried around to open the door I fumbled in my pockets for some coins for the fare. The cabbie looked at me and said not to bother and helped me out of the cab. As I thanked him and tried to get some money out of my pockets, my legs once again lost focus but fortunately the cabbie supported my weight. Given I am 6'4" and he was barely 5'10" I felt terrible and rather embarrassed as he helped me to the A&E reception window. They asked for my name and for my date of birth and with that he helped me into one of the seats in the waiting area. I tried to thank him again and pay him, but he insisted that he was fine and made sure once again that I was ok before departing. It is those types of acts that raise the bar for humanity as a whole and keep us striving to be better. Those of us that despite the constant barrage of shitty acts carried out by petty shitty people, keep the faith and act accordingly. I was always moved by the words that evil happens when good men fail to act, or something like that. It always meant to me that we have the ability to create heaven or hell here on earth by our own simple choice on whether to be a good man who acts or be a good man in name only. It seems to me nowadays we have plenty of good people in name only and few who are prepared to act. I was just in the presence of one of those good men who backed it up with action and for that if you ever read this, thank you. It also meant that I must look as bad as I felt, and I felt like absolute shit.

As I moaned hunched forward trying to hold together my gut which now felt like a washing machine filled with rocks and broken glass, I suddenly found I was confronted by a young girl just as I was saying to myself how much this fucking hurt. Note to self, stop saying what you're feeling. This young girl who was there with her family must have been around 5 years old, looked me straight in the eye and said "Mommy, is this man going to be alright? He doesn't look very good" As her parents quickly grabbed her hand and yanked her away, I thought it was now official, I did look like shit. As my name was called, two medical staff helped me into a wheelchair. I thought to myself, out of the mouths of babes and fools comes the truth and the little girl had nailed it and I also wondered "Mommy was I going to be alright?"

Now I had been to the A&E before with a problematic gastric ulcer and certain other gastric problems over the past 12 months and all the previous occasions before had resulted in me being prodded, pressed, probed and asked the same questions at least 3 times by different people. So have you taken any pain killers, "Yes I have" "Which ones" "Some co-codamol", "How did you find they worked" "well they worked initially but lately not so much and that is why I am here" "How many did you take" "Quite a few as I recall, and when they didn't work I came here" "We need to know exactly how many you took" "I think I took 8" "Over what time period" "I don't know, the last couple of hours since my guts have been killing me". With experience I found the right answer to all questions like this was "The prescribed dose". If you deviate from this you are liable to end up having a discussion with someone about how many, when exactly with them calmly asking you while you are having your insides turned inside out. As frustrating as this questioning process is, it usually ends with "I think we should give him some more paracetamol and codeine" which is what I was taking before I got here and if it had worked, I wouldn't be here. It was my second time in the A&E after several scans and prods by quite a few doctors. "Does it hurt if I push here" "Yes it hurts" "Does it hurt if I push here and release?" "Yes, that hurts, it actually fucking hurts, does that fact that I am convulsing, sweating like a pig, using English words like, fuck this fucking hurts give you a clue as to what I might be experiencing". After a series of examinations like this I remember one female doctor coming in and after relatively few jabs announcing she had seen my scan and that since I was experiencing serious abdominal pain, "Please give him 50 ml of Morphine Phosphate". With that a small plastic syringe was shoved into my mouth and a rather bitter fluid was pumped down the back of my throat. As I tried to get the bitter taste out of my mouth, suddenly something miraculous happened, the washing machine full of broken glass and fishhooks on a spin cycle that was my stomach, suddenly all the glass and fishhooks turned into salted caramel and the spin went to a gentle wash cycle.

This all happened in a space of 10 seconds. I immediately wanted to marry this woman for she was an angel sent to save me from the tortures that had befallen me. Thank you so much I said to her, reaching out to hold her hand and complete the human connection. My angel of a doctor looked at me and said "So glad that worked but we will want to keep you for a while to monitor you" "Anything you say", I responded as I would have married her if she had wanted at that moment. As I felt better it suddenly occurred to me I needed to find out what I had been given, "What was I just given?" "Morphine Phosphate 50ml" said one of the nurses, "how long will this last or has this just fixed me?" "No, it's just a pain killer and it varies from individual to individual" said the nurse..

The only previous experience I had ever had with Morphine had been many years previous. I had a very endearing friend who was a Model who had been in an accident and was very medicated. She in fact used to like to share her Morphine Lollipops with me. I never really thought much of them at the time so I didn't expect that much. The trick I found out to taking Morphine is to be in excruciating pain before you take it, and in excruciating pain fortunately I was. So after receiving the morphine, given that I had been in agonizing pain for hours and was exhausted, I promptly fell asleep. My body just crashed. I slept soundly for a few hours until I was awoken by a nurse asking if she could take my vitals which meant blood pressure, pulse, blood oxygenation and temperature. As I woke, again I became aware of the pain in my stomach, as she asked me to move the pain got worse. I asked if I could have more morphine. She said not at the moment but she could give me some paracetamol. "Why did you wake me up? When you knew how much pain I had been in if you knew you could not give me more morphine, why would you do that?" "Well we need to take your vitals every 4 hours" "Thanks a lot" I said, "If you could inform the Doctor that I am now up again and in excruciating pain and surprise, surprise my blood pressure is a little high and I am requesting some more morphine, I am not feeling well at all." "I will tell her when I see her," said my nurse. With that she walked off as if I had just ruined her evening. As the wash cycle containing fish hooks and glass that was my stomach started to speed up I wondered what sort of hell had I found myself in and made a mental note to ignore all further requests from that nurse.

My experience with these gastric flare ups had taught me that once they start that I was in for at least 18-24 hours of gut wrenching pain. The gut wrenching, wishing I was dead, no comfortable positions, type of pain where there was nothing else to do but wait it out. I had tried so many different things to block out this type of pain, from meditations to using electro stim machines. Nothing seemed to work apart from good old

Morphine Phosphate. I had investigated trying to get hold of some of those Morphine Lollipops that I had underappreciated so many years ago but alas this was impossible as Morphine is a restricted drug.

As a side note During the First World War, department stores, including Harrods, sold kits containing syringes, needles and tubes of cocaine and heroin. It was promoted as a present for friends on the frontline – shoot up to make life in the trenches more bearable and alleviate the horrors of war.

Now I do understand why we have drug laws and certain drugs are restricted and not freely available. I always find it interesting that in 1900 here in London one could purchase pharmaceutical grade cocaine hydrochloride from any drugstore without a prescription. It was sold in a tin that came with a syringe for injecting it. I also found it amusing that the way to offer a Victorian lady some cocaine was not to offer her a line but a vein, the best way for cocaine to be appreciated was to inject it into a vein in one's upper thigh. I was thinking of how hard it was for the young men of that time to deliver that line with a straight face. Given the many layers of clothes that had to come off to give the lady some cocaine. I can imagine a young man saying that it wasn't up to him but if she wanted to try some of his cocaine the only way that one can take it is to inject it into one's upper thigh, so all your clothes have to come off. Sorry but that's the only way to take it, I promise I won't look. Whoever came up with that one, his name seems to be lost in history. It's stories like that that make me wonder how much we have really evolved in the last hundred years. For all the talk you hear about those prudish Victorians, you could get cocaine at every corner drug store, theatres encouraged the audience to meet the actors and actresses, and if all else failed you also had the odd opium den. Mr Selfridge of Selfridges fame died a pauper after getting involved with twin sisters that had a love of gambling and cocaine. The Hell Fire club in High Wycombe, and we like to think we are all that. I have never seen a girl ask for a line of cocaine, strip before the line was even laid out, just a regular Tuesday for a Victorian. It really makes you think how much edge pushing we really do nowadays or do we just like to think we do.

What I did know was that once these gastric episodes started, I had two choices. I could either lie on the sofa at home moaning, wishing for death or to get myself to the CW A&E and spend my time there hoping to get a few hours reprieve from time to time from Mr Morphine. Also during these flare ups my blood pressure would often go to 220 over 140 and at 180 they are supposed to send you to hospital. I felt I had a valid reason to be there.

Let me say I have had some experience with pain. I suffered a herniated disc a few years before and I have endured back surgeries that had definitely made me aware of what it was like to live with serious pain. I am experienced with the use of painkillers such as dihydrocodeine and I had tramadol before I had surgery for my herniated disc. I still remember the first time that I had been given morphine phosphate but the one thing that I don't understand is why anyone would ever want to take morphine recreationally. I remember years ago sucking on Morphine Lollipops with a highly medicated, double jointed, model friend and apart from her engaging company being completely underwhelmed by these morphine lollipops. I recall not really feeling much of anything until I realized the secret to what the wow factor of Morphine was. You firstly must be in agonizing pain to appreciate the wow factor. for me I don't see how this could be a fun recreational drug. Maybe for abusive couples who like to beat the shit out of each other, generally inflict, Morphine is the most amazing make up drug. Unfortunately, I didn't find morphine alleviates any sort of emotional pain or frustration caused by stupid insensitive people asking redundant questions. This last visit to the hospital has allowed me to test that thoroughly so we are only talking about physical pain. So two guys wanting to get off on Morphine on a Friday night would first have to kick each other in the balls a few times to get the ball rolling. Then once agonizing pain had been reached by both, a few shots of Morphine and you could experience the "Oh my God my balls don't hurt anymore sensation". I just am not seeing the pay off.

Still till this day the events of that Thursday are a bit blurred, but here is what I remember. When I was first admitted, the examination area next to mine contained several people surrounding one other man who had been admitted and they all seemed to be talking Turkish or something like it. At least one of those languages where the rules dictate that if 3 or more people are gathered a minimum of two must be talking at full volume at all times for the conversation to be valid. Since there seemed to be around 5 this meant that 3 seemed to be the number that needed to be talking at full volume at the same time. I remember thinking that at least they would drown out my moaning and groans of pain. I responded as clearly as I could to the questions I was asked by all the Doctors and nurses that examined me. "Where does it hurt?" "It hurts in my stomach." "Does it hurt if I tap?" "Yes it hurts when you tap" "Does it hurt more if I push and release or if I just push?" "It hurts both ways, I am sorry it just really hurts, I have been here before and I took Co-Codomol before I got here which wasn't working, which is why I came here, can I get something stronger for the pain as it really hurts?" "How much did you take?" "The prescribed amount". "Ok we can look into that for you" said the Doctor. I always liked when they used the royal we in that sense, like they would form a pain quorum with their colleagues to decide how best to treat this man's pain dilemma. To me this just meant, no time soon.

As the pain started to come in waves, I made my case a little stronger saying that the pain was quite bad and if they didn't give me something for the pain my groans were at risk of disturbing the Turkish support group. Once again, a Doctor came to my bedside "Do you mind if I examine you?" "No, I don't mind if you examine me, I thought you would never ask" "Does it hurt if I tap here?" "Yes" "Does it hurt if I press here?" "Yes actually" "What about now?" "Fuck yes it hurts" I really started to wonder if during these Doctors' medical training they ever mentioned looking for secondary indicators of pain like eyes rolling, clutching at ones stomach, requests from the patient to be "Knocked the fuck out", If Dexter, the TV based serial killer, forensic scientist who only kills bad people, seems to do it with a quick syringe to the neck for the love of God just Dexter me! "I think we need a scan" was the response, "Are you kidding me? Can I please have some pain killers before I go to get scanned? Please!!" "We can certainly look at that" "Fuck you!! and no I don't want any paracetamol." "Nurse, can we get him some pain killers" "Hello so I hear you are in pain, I have some codeine for you" It is at this point that I have to assume it's a slow day on the comedy channel in heaven and that God was getting his kicks tormenting me for laughs" Jesus Christ, have you not had enough laughs today, please Lucifer just take me know. Not that I am religious, but from all my reading and understanding of what it takes to get into heaven, if I end up there there has definitely been a huge administrative error and not to mention that most of my experiences with others on earth including some in the A&E would mean that I wouldn't know anyone if I went to heaven anyway. So Lucifer, who I often thought got a very rough deal from the almighty, and as I am part of God's creation, I wouldn't kneel before me or most of the other individuals that make up mankind. For that one action his punishment is he gets to rule in hell. Given that he started out as an ArchAngel, it always sounded like he got railroaded by God to me.

Given they say that a big part of medicine is the power of observation, when a patient constantly asks to be knocked out, struggles to control the muscle spasms from chronic pain, has told you he has been this way for a few hours, the fact that this is taking place in a modern city, in a modern hospital and not some red cross tent in the Gaza strip one would think that the response "We have some codeine and paracetamol for you" is the stuff of Monty Python. I also imagine they had, "Jesus loves you and is praying you feel better" in their arsenal of pain relief. Where the fuck is John Cleese when you need him, someone should be writing this down

As I recall when finally, my suffering had no more comedic value for the gods on high I was rewarded by having a syringe of Morphine Phosphate pumped into my mouth as my gurney was pushed off for me to get yet another scan. God I hope this morphine lasts. I remember thinking that my gut felt like the inside of a spin dryer tumbling fish hooks, glass and rocks and the spin cycle was on high. Yes that is how it felt, fucking diabolically bad, please knock me out was the over riding thought that kept running through my mind. Dexter made it look so easy, I must find out what he uses and ask if they had some. Fuck this hurts.

Magnetic Resonance Imaging (MRI) is a non-invasive way to take a look at what's going on inside someone's body. It uses a magnetic field and radio waves to alter the hydrogen atoms in your body. When they realign themselves, a radio signal is emitted, what is captured is interpreted by a computer to produce a 2D or 3D image of the scanned area. This image is examined by a radiologist and given to your doctor to aid in your diagnosis. Then there is a Contrast MRI. In some cases, your doctor may request advanced MRI services with contrast. This is a liquid dye solution that is injected into your veins and because of how it travels through magnetic fields. shows your insides with greater resolution. As the contrast makes its way into your system, most patients will notice a very warm feeling that spreads throughout their body for about 20 seconds during and after the injection. This is often concentrated around the groin area and you might think that you are passing urine, but you are not. What they don't tell you is that the warm feeling feels like warm liquid diarrhea swirling around your stomach and when you expect it to stop around your nether regions it doesn't and it feels like you have just let all that diarrhea just leak out of your ass and the warm feeling you feel in your legs is the warm diarrhea as it makes its way down the back of your legs. They also don't seem to take into account that you are practically naked and for some reason there is always a group of at least 3 or 4 people hanging around in a scan room. You are also usually pretty much naked. So when it feels like your anal sphincter has just given up and let all that warm diarrhea flow all down your legs the operator then asks you to remain still while the machine tells you to take a deep breath and hold it. One is left wondering if it is to save yourself from what must be the god awful smell that is about to sweep over you. The machine then tells you to breathe normally. As you are ejected from the machine and the odd nurse or health care assistant comes around you, your hands reach down expecting to be immersed in the flood of liquid shit that you have just left on the table. You notice the non plus looks on the faces of the young nurses and scan technicians as you expect some type of response to you shitting all over their machine. Nothing, so you are naked and covered in your own shit and nothing on their faces. Has their job so jaded them that your performance at this Chelsea scat party is deemed unimpressive. As I came out of the scanner, all sense of pride and common decency had gone as I felt around expecting to grasp handfuls of my own shit to find nothing. I wrapped my gown around my ready to be moved back on to the gurney again with some weird sense of pride. I was still a man, I just endured a scan, not a passive gimp at some chelsea late night scat party for scan technicians. One of the nurses lent over to me and asked "Are you in pain" "Yes I am" in so many ways I thought. As my gurney was pushed back up to the A&E the fish hooks grabbed at my gut once again but at least I hadn't sprayed the bed with shit, so that was a positive.

As I was returned to the A&E ward there was a flurry of Doctors all wanting to tap me, prod me, push me, all asking me if it hurt. I vaguely remember getting back to the point when I was pleading with them all to please knock me out, "Please Dexter me, just do it please! It hurts so much". Yes I sort of recall going into full wimp mode, even crying a bit while moaning for the pain to stop. To any woman reading this I totally concede, especially at that moment, I was a whining little bitch incapable of what it takes to give birth to a child. I want to get out in front and admit this straight away. I am sure as a man I make up for it in other ways, I am also aware that the information on how we as men actually make up for it has currently been misplaced due to a filing error. "We need you to sign a consent form" "Can I please have some morphine?" "Yes you can have some morphine" " I will sign anything if I can please have some Morphine. Thank you, thank you, did I mention it's ok to knock me out if you want" with that, I believe I signed my consent form for surgery. As morphine was syringed into my mouth, once again I passed out to the sound of my own moaning. "Thank you, Dexter, you beautiful soul for hearing my prayer" and that is all I can remember.

Chapter 2

Can I take your Vitals, life on the SMA

As I came too, I found myself on the Post Operative care ward St Mary Abbot or the SMA as it is known to the staff. Someone mentioned it was Friday and it seemed that I had somehow lost Thursday. I felt as if I had been beaten, my guts sliced open, I found that I was attached to bags of unspeakable body fluids that I came to realize flowed from me. A few litres of bright orange urine connected to a bag connected to my penis; mine, a bag of green slimy shit, attached to a tube exiting from my right side; mine, another bag best described as blood mixed with pus attached to a tube exiting my left side; also mine. All this coupled with a searing case of the worst indigestion known to man, just fucking shoot me and then as if in a sketch from footlights a nurse approached my bed "how are you feeling and can I take your vitals". Thinking that this person looked like a nurse and was there to render care I said " I am in a lot of pain and feel terrible" "Can I take your vitals" she asked "Yes Ok, can I get something for the pain" "As soon as I have your vitals I will get you some paracetamol and codeine." This again, welcome to hell I thought, at least I was finally here.

In the NHS for some reason, it has been chiselled in stone that every 4 hours no matter who you are, what you are there for, no matter if you were in terrible agony and are now sleeping, enjoying being unconscious and not writhing in pain, NHS caregivers will wake you from your slumber to ask if they can take your vitals. The funny thing is that you can refuse which really pisses them off even if waking you really pisses you off. They are like Gammas in Aldous Huxley's Brave New World, there to collect vitals and get very upset if they don't get to perform their function. "He won't allow me to collect his vitals", "but he is dead", "fucking selfish patients".

Vital signs, i.e. respiratory rate, oxygen saturation, pulse, blood pressure and temperature, are regarded as an essential part of monitoring hospitalized patients. Changes in vital signs prior to clinical deterioration are well documented and early detection of preventable outcomes is key to timely intervention. NHS 15 Jan 2019

It turns out that I had woken up Friday evening after stumbling in just after midnight Thursday morning and from the looks and feel of things I had an operation that I believe had lasted a few hours. My gown felt a tad small and given I was 6'4 it seemed someone had chosen a medium for me. As I rolled around groaning in my postoperative delirium I now understood how models backstage at fashion shows get so blasé. At some point when you get prodded, pushed, poked, examined, talked about as if you're not there, the concept of nudity disappears. You are a skin bag containing a commodity that for some reason someone values. For patients the system is trying to render you well so it can discharge you and take in the next unwell skin bag, for models they are the best autonomous coat hangers that money can buy. You can see how models harbour such self-loathing especially for the guys that want to fuck them. You want to fuck this autonomous coat hanger, your fucking weird, I am just going to do it because it feels good and for a second I can believe I am not here with you. As a patient, this is the thought process when a nurse tries to cover your genitals with an undersized gown, it is like your care about this body while you have stuck a catheter up its penis that the owner can't feel, attached to a bag with 3 liters of his own piss, given it enemas until it drips shit, have not changed the dressings on the holes you made to extract all this horrible shit and now you want to act like you care about its dignity by covering the penis on display. Give me some pain medication so I can drift off and make believe I am not here. So, I suppose this is an example of how you can link sex with models to Morphine for patients. As it turns out I would be a hopeless heroin addict or at least a very frustrated one as it is incredibly hard to spike a vein in my arm. This was shown to be true as I had catheter champions asked to come down to try and put a working catheter in me. The frustrated nurse after numerous attempts then list a quick list of pills that she was about to give me to which I replied "I am in a lot of fucking pain and no I don't mind if you try to spike my vein later" She then also mentioned the magic M word. After the pills and what I really hoped was apple juice as there seemed a lot of containers filled with my urine were hanging around, she then pushed a plastic syringe of magic M into my mouth and suddenly I was off to a better place, fuck God as once again I didn't have to make deals for my soul for pain relief, I had done a deal with Mr Morphine.

I feel at this point I must once again say that Morphine is only great if you feel fucking awful to start of with, excruciating pain type I found is best. Anyone reading this I can assure you that this drug from my perspective has no recreational value and I would not recommend an abusive relationship as a gateway opportunity either.

In my case I just mentally escaped the post operative ward of St Mary Abbot to a world where my penis didn't have a foot long tube extending into it, my own unspeakable bodily fluids openly collecting in bags and where my stomach had not exploded spraying all its vile fluid everywhere, only to be hosed down and sewn up like an old leather duffel. I was off to a softer place with my friend Mr Morphine, and I really do not care if you take my vitals or not. When I next woke the nurse informed me that I had been connected to an automatic morphine dispensing machine. All I now had to do was to hit the little green button when it shone a green light and a shot of morphine would be released into my system through the intravenous cannula connected to my forearm. This did indeed sound interesting. Green light button shining, ok, push, go, a quick beep and then I lay back and suddenly the fish hooks inside my gut didn't seem to be so noticeable. No green light, Nurse? "Well once you press the button you have to wait 5 minutes before you can press it again, otherwise." "Yeah yeah I get it too much of a good thing, in this place the danger was a nasty case of RSI of the thumb, I asked "how much longer?" "Four minutes, 30 seconds", said the nurse. Ok this seems like a good idea, I always felt that I never suffered from an addictive personality. This should be just the ticket, how much longer nurse, can you check? "4 minutes, 10 seconds to go", she said. " So what am I supposed to do while I am waiting?" "I can take your vitals," said the nurse. "Ok then". I offered my limbs willingly as I waited to pass the time as quickly as possible. Blood pressure, temperature, pulse, all ok. "So nurse have you got everything? This green light hasn't come back on yet?" "2 minutes 20 seconds to go" said the nurse. For fucks sake, I thought. "It's definitely working right?" "Yes", said the nurse, "Your urine is looking fairly dark, you should drink more water" she said "I will" as I looked at her with my green light still not on face. "1 minute, I think I am going to empty your urine bag" she said. "Knock yourself out" I said. Still no fucking green light. What the fuck then suddenly green light came on, right make sure the catheter in my arm is at the right angle. Houston I have a green light here, I pushed the button again and this time I made sure that my catheter was perfectly angled for maximum throughput and away we went. Mr Morphine took me by the hand and suddenly chocolate fish hooks instead of steel and slow wash cycle rather than spin. The virtual stomach slash wound now gone, "All better now" said the nurse in a condescending tone. Fuck you I thought, the Harpy had been denied dining on my delicious misery, she would now have to go a find some other patient torment. "I am fine now thanks" she rolled her eyes and walked away, I had a direct line to Mr Morphine now so screw her. I thought to myself how certain types of nurses such as the Harpy I currently had, must absolutely hate it when patients have weapons they can use against their power to make their patients miserable. They must consider it almost blasphemous and against the rules of the game. Misery and pain was theirs to administer, how dare the patients think that they had some control over their recovery, their bodies, they ran the wards, it was their territory, and now I had gone against the tide. I now had a weapon to fight back the pain monster and its minions were not happy. I was no longer prey and I was going to work out how to survive in this ecosystem.

As I finally came too again it was Saturday evening. I had spent the last 24 hours riding through a dream-like state of having my gut caught on fish hooks only to have them all turn to salted caramel fish hooks as I destroyed them with my green button blaster. Slowly surfacing I looked around the confines of my bed I thought it a good time to take stock of things, tubes, bag of blood, bag of green shit, couple liters of bright orange urine connected to a tube disappearing up my penis, green button machine carrying my buddy Mr M and the dubious connection to my vein through the on again, off again catheter, everything was here. I then remembered that I just had a secondary phone that had a sim card with no credit and no banking apps and unfortunately about 5% charge. I must make contact with the outside world, I thought. I checked and I had a total of £60 cash, 3 £20 notes and some pound coins. I had my leather satchel I came in with which had my pants inside, no shirt anywhere, a pair of vans shoes, no keys (I can find out what happened to them later) , and my glasses , thank God.

I surveyed my room which happened to contain 5 other occupants. The man opposite me had cancer and seemed to be married to a woman who reminded me of Winnie Mandella which softened my heart when I saw how much she fussed over him, even after he had sternly told her to stop. The man to my left who I will refer to as Sir Percivil as he was in his 70's, spoke in a loud booming cut glass english accent and was slightly deaf as far as I could tell. As the evening drew closer the pain in my stomach reminded me that this cannula was not really optimal and that I needed some Oral Morphine to stop the pain cycle switching from wash to spin. The next thing I heard was Sir Percivil's booming voice announcing the following "There is a stool in my anus that is causing me discomfort and it should be removed!" and again "There is a stool in my anus that is causing me discomfort and needs to be removed!!". As one of the young black nurses seemed to come to his aid asking what seemed to be the trouble, he asked her to come closer and said he didn't want anyone else to hear so she could draw the privacy curtain. He then proceeded to say in the loudest of voices that she needed to remove this troublesome stool from his anus but she must apply generous amounts of cream to his anus after it is removed and she must have the cream ready. No one else in the room should know. Everyone in the room looked around wondering where to look. The man on my right had the sweetest of wives who I believe was Caroline, he unfortunately had the onset of Parkinson's and I could see the strain on Caroline's face. She looked like the very epitome of the perfect dutiful Hampshire village wife. Quite a looker in her day she now had silver hair, was in her mid 60's and had lived her life supporting her husband and following her wedding vowels. You could see that the ordeal was weighing on her. You could tell that coming to London where all these crazy people were to support her husband in this big hospital not far from the infamous Kings Road, she was trying her best to be the supportive wife that she always was, you could imagine Caroline as an active member of her local parish helping the church raise money by baking things. She was just not used to all of this. As Sir Percival bellowed to his nurse to apply generous amounts of cream to his anus as the troublesome stool had now been removed. Then Sir Percival said something priceless. As an extra large dollop of cream was applied to his anus he cried out praise the Lord and what I can only imagine was some public school mantra he said. "Praise be to God for the Lord said to the boy that he must love thy father" "Oh my God more, Praise be to God for the Lord said to the boy that he must love thy father" with everyone else outside the curtain not knowing where to look, I caught Caroline's eye and she covered her mouth and closed her eyes and held her husband's hand, it was all a bit much. Later I saw her chatting with Winnie, the black wife of the man opposite me and I imagined Caroline back in her village recounting the events of the day about the man and the cream on his anus and how she even now had a black female friend which I imagined may have been her first. All I can say is that the look on Carolines face was priceless, as every loud mention of anus made her nervously giggle, look at her husband and hold his hand even tighter. I thought how lucky he was to be loved by such a devoted woman, it was nice to think love and devotion like that still exists. The final chap across diagonally from me I had heard had been some sort of musical creative genius before he was not and lay in the corner bed sulking, his short frame rarely covered by anything, his head would pop up from the sheets every so often, reminding me of Uncle Fester with his dark sullen eyes and bald head. He was tended to be a personal nurse that was changed every 12 hours and when he was offered a spoon of food or wanted to say something and his carer lent over to hear his murmur often resulting in him spitting on his carer, the carer would then reply "John, it's not nice to spit on me" "John is a not being a very nice boy" John's name was repeatedly called out by his carers. "Would John like this?" , "John, just one more mouthful?", "John don't spit at me you naughty boy". I always wanted to find out what health plan he was on but no one, not even the nurses seemed to know, they didn't even seem to know why he was there.

They constantly tried to keep him within the confines of his bed but every now and again he would kick out with his feet often landing a decent body blow which they replied with "now John is being a bit naughty".

When John wanted to further show his dissatisfaction with his care staff he would throw off the sheet covering him and urinate over whoever was not quick enough to respond. I remember hearing one nurse say "he is doing it again" while the older black female carer replied "Why is John spraying himself everywhere like that". Over the next few days as far as I could tell across the room they were looking after a version of Uncle Fester with a concealed urine pistol. As far as I could tell John, who one night played born free on his phone for 2 hours until everyone in the room yelled at him to stop, basically suffered from being a congenital arsehole.

As things then quietened down and I managed to get my cannula lined up properly again, Sir Percival's words crossed my mind as I green buttoned myself away from the scene, being bent over while have a troublesome stool removed by some young nurse only to have his ass covered with big dollops of soothing cream. After all I had been through the last few days it didn't sound that bad to me at all. Lucky bastard, I thought, he definitely is in control of his ecosystem, I should take note and do the same. What is my version of a big dollop of cool cream on my anus? With that thought my mind drifted away. The wash cycle that was my stomach shifted to gentle and the

tubes that at times seemed to tug on my

balls let up and with that I drifted off to

sleep.

Chapter 3

Things that scream in the night

"Let me out of here, I am going to call the Police, do not touch me!! You can't touch me, call the police, HELP!, HELP! I know my rights, get your hands off me you pervert" These were the words that yanked me out of my slumber at 2.00am Sunday morning. What was happening, who was being assaulted? When she first came into view as she made her way down the ward, I saw she had long gray hair, no teeth to speak of and was fending off the black male nurse that was in her way, using her zimmer frame as a battering ram. It turned out that

Bea liked to indulge in a few late night cigarettes outside and she would not be denied. The only way I can describe the voice I heard is to imagine the Wicked Witch of the East chain smoking for 40 years, having discovered immunity from lung cancer she was now being held hostage on our ward, the good old SMA (Saint Mary Abbot). It turned out she was quite famous and known as Screaming Bea of the SMA. Some wrinkles in the government's regulations, benefits, etc meant someone had admitted Beatrice for something a while ago, it could not have been dental since she had no teeth and not lung cancer since I believe she was close to 80 . The nursing home where she was from was now in a legal dispute with the hospital about taking her back. She now had made her home the ward of Saint Mary Abbot and be damned if anyone was going to remove her from her new home.

This is what woke me from my slumber at 2am on a Sunday as I lay in a bed in the same medium gown that I arrived in, with the same god awful bags of disgusting bodily fluids attached to tubes coming out of me. What was more, something didn't smell too good and me being yanked out of my slumber meant my stomach began to burn again. I clicked my green button, nothing, I then had to endure the long 5 minute wait until I could have another go. An eternity passed until the green light finally came on. Bang, I pushed the button, the fish hooks were still there but no nasty minions yanking on them, still this is not good. I have to catch someone's eye, press a buzzer, get some attention, please can I have some pain meds, "I will check with the nurse and let you know"said the nurse. "I really need them as I am in a lot of pain", "You have your automatic morphine dispenser you know"said the nurse. It seems a lot of the nursing staff seem to be taught that stating the obvious passes as a way of answering patients questions. No, I had not realized that the hand held green button connected to this machine was a pain dispenser, but now that you pointed it out things will be much better. The pain that I am experiencing that is forcing me to spasm and clutch my gut and pull this face will surely be fixed by you stating the obvious.

Yes I realize what my mechanical friend is for but the tube that connects the pain relieving morphine to me relies upon a clear pathway into my veins and given I am still in the same gown and I found myself in days ago, the fact that none of my dressing have been changed, the fact that to cannulate me properly has been such a challenge that nurses and doctors known to be good at this have paid me a visit to try their luck. As it turns out there may not be a clear path for the Morphine to make its way into my body via this second rate cannula that is trying its best just to hold on to my arm let alone provide an intravenous passage of medication."That rarely happens" is all she said. Oh great I thought, I was now almost certain that her appointment as a nurse had to be the result of affirmative action in the workplace. "Well I can assure you the pain is real, can I have some oral morphine please as I promise you it is hurting". With that she disappeared saying she would tell the other nurse. As I lay there clutching my gut, every now and again forgetting that a few feet of tube attached to my penis would catch something, giving it a good tug, which felt like it somehow was connected to a few of the fish hooks in my gut with a fine thread tied to my left testicle just to make life interesting. "How bad is your pain?" said the nurse as she approached my bed "How bad is my pain, how bad is my pain?" I am here with a crazy screaming lady, I have gut wrenching pain, a first-year medical student could see that my cannula could only be used as an example of how not to cannulate a patient. I have a tube inserted into my penis making me wonder if I will ever use it for anything remotely sexual as it felt more part of the external tube system than a part of my body. "The Pain is very fucking bad right now ok", "Just be patient, have you tried pressing your green button" "Are you kidding me yes it had occurred to me to press the green button but I think its blocked" " That rarely happens you know" "Please just give me some oral morphine to end this and put me out of my misery." "I will need to get sign off" said the nurse. "Please get it then" I said, wondering if I was once again being used by the gods for their comedic amusement. "Oh you need sign off and I am in excruciating pain with a faulty green button, on second thoughts if you have to go to the trouble of getting another minion to sign off on this to make sure you don't fuck up, do not bother, REALLY. They say the secret to being a good nurse is being observant. I heard a lot of nurse conversations about how their own observation skills often trumped young doctors in defining what was wrong with a patient. I would have been better off with a blind nurse for all the observational logic being utilized by this caregiver, and I use that term loosely. Once again I thought Lucifer, my old friend, just take me now since I am tired of my role in this divine comedy. As I lay there waiting for the Morphine that would release me from the clutch of this demonic Harpy of a nurse,

"There you go" said the nurse as she shoved the syringe in my mouth and released its pain relieving motherload. In less than a minute the steel fish hooks and tubes somehow connected to my left testicle would become salted caramel, dissolving and releasing me from their tyrannical grip. As I slipped away I could hear Bea in the background yelling "Leave me be, leave me be, let me alone Now!!" I found myself in agreement with Bea, leave me be you bunch of bastards and for the next hour Mr Morphine kept them at bay. I will deal with Mr Green Button malfunctioning in the morning., "Can I take your vitals?" said another nurse, which I thought was a tad redundant as at that point she could have taken my temperature with a broom handle up my arse and I would be powerless to stop her. "And here is your pain medicine", a squirt of Morphine, fuck yeah, didn't need you again God HAHA!!.

I drifted back into consciousness to Sir Percival's request for more cream to be applied to his anus. The way I was feeling I was starting to wonder if a big dollop of cool cream over my anus might be just the ticket. As I rolled over onto my back my collection of tubes suddenly dragged against my various openings including the tube in my penis and suddenly I was very aware it had been several hours since my pain medication. "Can I take your vitals," said the nurse, "can you lift your arm up?" "No not really but if you get me my pain medication to go with my pressing my little green button we might have a deal.

As I was to find out that having a fully functioning cannula really is the secret to the auto analgesic dispenser and having crap veins ruled out me ever having a decent appreciation for heroin, the auto morphine green button experience was on and off depending on the quality of the cannula that was being used. I was later to be blessed by a visit from a true medical professional called Dr Tom whose cannula would have turned the green button into a high quality Yale door lock to the land of Mr Morphine rather than a shoddy Chinese knock off lock that some times worked and sometimes left me stranded on the wrong side of the door with a stomach full of fish hooks.

Chapter 4

Savaged by the Beast

Sunday passed with me drifting in and out of sleep, depending on whether my gut was on spin cycle or wash cycle and whether I was getting my morphine assists every 4 hours along with my potential access to Mr Morphine via the green button. Monday morning came and along with it a visit from a representative from the pain team, one of which I vaguely remember meeting over the weekend to explain the green button to me. It was now time to take me off the machine and given the lock to the door was increasingly becoming Chinese knock off as opposed to decent Yale lock I was in agreement. I told the representative from the pain team that I was concerned that I would have access to the oral morphine as I knew how long it was effective for and how long it took to act. He told me that along with the oral morphine they were also going to introduce me to Tramadol 50mg on a 4 per day cycle. So oral morphine 50ml would be given on a 4 hour cycle and the Tramadol 50mg 4 times per day. Ok that seemed reasonable and we agreed that I would be taken off the machine that afternoon. Around 3pm that afternoon I was disconnected from the machine and managed to secure a syringe of morphine and a Tramadol tablet to see me off. As it turned out, before my hospital admission I had been talking to someone about working for them on a tech project and all of a sudden I received a message that they wanted a call at 8pm. As it happened I also had a visitor who was going to bring me my computer at last, up until that time I had only had a second rate phone without any banking apps and only access to the slowest of hospital wifi. My friend arrived with my laptop and immediately I felt a little more connected. As I thanked my friend I became slightly aware of the fact that I was still wearing the same gown that I had woken up in last Friday and the fact that my penis was mostly on display as it felt more like one of the tubes the hung from my body rather than a body part as he kept mentioning that he didn't need to see my balls. I kept trying to arrange myself and it was only when one of the nurses was taking my vitals that she mentioned my gown was looking a little dirty and it was strange that I was wearing a medium one. "A medium one I thought, I am 6 '4 and weigh 120 kg and someone thought medium. I just thought that the hospital staff liked access when it seemed that an individual had decided that I bare most of my bits to the world. Whoever you were, great choice. "Would you like another gown in a larger size?" "Yes please," I said, " becoming more aware of my disheveled state. By around 6,30pm all this activity had led to my stomach full of fish hooks to start to go from a slow manageable wash cycle to a threatening intermittent spin cycle. As the last dose of pain meds had been given to me at 3pm I asked to see my nurse who of course said to be safe that I would not be able to have my next dose of pain meds until 8pm. This would happen from time to time when a nurse would just decide that 4 hours would start from whenever she thought. Now I had to sort of be on point for a call at 8pm but given that she was one of the bitch Harpy type nurses as opposed to a normal human caregiver, I could tell that 8pm would be my only chance at pain relief. Fortunately my friend who was visiting me was one of those creative, healing, empathetic types and could sense my frustration at the response from the bitch harpy nurse and her resolve to only give me the pain relief at 8pm. So as 7pm passed my stomach full of fish hooks upped the ante by switching to a slow spin cycle.

"Things will be fine" my friend told me,"Just

breath and don't think about the pain, as I

focussed on his calm voice, it was like

throwing sponges into the wash that dulled

the edges of the fish hooks. It was then

around 7.40pm that the nurse popped by to

say that she wanted my vitals. I told her that

I was in pain and she responded telling me

that she was preparing my pain meds. As I

shifted to allow her to take my blood

pressure and temperature it was like a cup

full of nails just got thrown into the wash. My

friend told me to relax and offered me his

hand which I took and tried to focus on his

calming voice not to think about the pain. As

I focused as hard as I could, the spin cycle

started to accelerate. What was the time?

7.50pm. I can get the pain meds, sort my head out and be late for the call as the calls with this chap did always seem to start a little late. "Don't think about the pain, the nurse is getting your meds now, no need to worry" "No need to worry I thought as I could hold on for another few minutes. Over the next few minutes the spin cycle switched from regular spin to ultra dry spin and I grabbed my friend's hand with everything I had as I felt now like some of the fish hooks were connected to my testicles and every now and again one would be given a sharp tug. "The nurse is coming now" said my friend as she approached the bed. "How is the pain she asked" "What the fuck do you think I said?" "Wayne means it is quite bad" said my friend. "Yes it is quite bad, I followed up by saying" thinking to myself that I was actually due my pain meds at 7 pm. Raising the fact that it was her arbitrary decision to turn a 4 cycle into a 5 hour one I realised wouldn't be helpful. "I cant give it to you at the moment" she said, "Why the fuck not" I said", I need sign off" she said. You didn't think to get that during the last hour. "I have to be sure you need it" "You have to be fucking kidding me" and with that I felt the monster bite down into my gut. I was being presided over by one of the arch bitch Harpy minions and she was feeding on my pain and I was in her clutches. Even though my friend told me not to imagine the pain his voice was in the distance and it felt like I was in the presence of one of the Crazy 88 from Kill Bill, one of the timbers from the roof had fallen on me and trapped me and one of the Crazy 88 was slashing at my gut and hysterically laughing as he did it. Rather than the nurse looking like Lucy Lui she had the demeanor and look of Kathy Bates. So I was James Cann strapped to the bed in pain, holding onto my friend's hand, pleading for a little human understanding while the nurse Kathy Bates teased at providing me pain relief. As I gasped for air, aware that I was making a bit of a scene, she returned only to tell me that she couldn't give me the oral morphine as the computer was slow and that she had to wait for it. I was obviously dealing with the demon Kathy Bates herself, empathy was something that only other people had, appreciation for the human condition, something other people had, interest in care to anyone other than herself, once again something that only held back other people. As I lay there in the bed the spin cycle in my gut switched to full and with each spin it felt like a piece of my testicles were being caught up. The masked member of the Crazy 88 was slicing at my gut with all the precision of a master swordsman. Where the fuck wss Uma Thurman in all of this, at least if I was going to die. did I really have to die at the hands of insane Nurse Kathy Bates rather than a svelte Lucy Luu. I realized that my friend's voice was way off in the distance that I had lost all awareness for where I was as I held on for dear life. "Please make it stop" I said "just make him stop, please" All in all the dose of pain medication that was to release me from this torture arrived at 8.30pm.

Thirty minutes might not sound like a long

time but you get trapped under a fallen roof

beam, have your gut exposed, whipped with

fish hooks and then have it sliced repeatedly

by an expert swordsman turning my gut into

fine sashimi while crazy Kathy Bates looks

on, try it and you will see it is quite a long

time. When the syringe finally got shoved

into my mouth I felt myself resurface in the

bed, slightly aware that I may have

damaged my friend's hand as I had been

holding it for dear life, through the ordeal

and that I was now in the fetal position. I

was a damp, smelly mess as I had been

sweating profusely and was still in the same

gown and bed sheets that I had awoken in

the previous Friday and now it was Monday

night. As I became aware of my surroundings once again. I mumbled words of thanks and appreciation for without his support I felt it would have been far worse than it was. I jumped on the call for a quick 10 min minutes towards the end of the hour, thank god for those situations that are predictably late. I had just been savaged by the NHS post operative beast while one of its Harpy caregivers oversaw the execution of the savagery. I was alive and I was determined that I was going to survive. My friend stayed with me until 9.30pm, full 30 minutes after visiting hours as Kathy Bates was to remind us. To this day I am still so grateful for his presence during this episode. I now started to think how am I going to make it through this.

Later that night I worked out a plan that had the Harpy Nurse Kathy Bates cornered. The doctors had prescribed that I be on a 4 hour pain meds cycle as per my request I found out and I made sure I got my request in every chance I got. Her only shot back was that since she had administered the pain medicine at 8.30pm that I was not to have any further pain meds until 12.30 and boy I was watching those minutes like a hawk. It was weird, even though the sensation of having a member of the Crazy 88 slash me to pieces, it was all in my head. It felt like I had sustained the wound that was now in the process of healing. It had an almost Marvel Movie quality about it. In reality if it had really happened, I would be a very dead decomposing body right now, but in the Marvel SuperHero Universe I had survived the encounter and was healing, even Thor took moments to lick his wounds. At 12.20 I pressed my alarm to make sure that Kathy Bates was aware of my request and sensing the almighty scene I was going to create and given that she had lost support of the room by her actions, my pain meds were delivered to me on the dot of 12.30 including one 50mg Tramadol tablet. As Mr Morphine took my hand and turned all the fish hooks once again into salted caramel my stomach was now a salted caramel milkshake on a gentle spin cycle. As the pain ebbed away for the first time, I don't know how long it took but I suddenly felt hungry. I had been on a fluids only diet so water and apple juice had been my only sustenance for the last few days. I had survived being savaged by the beast, I had survived and had prevailed. Now I was going to hunt for calories as I had heard a rumor of a vending machine close by.

I reached into my treasure chest and removed one £20 bill and with the few coins I had with me, I put it all in a cup. There was then the matter of my two bags of bodily fluids, the first pusy blood bag and the second green fibrous bile bag, I found a medical zip tie and secured these two together and then in a nurses tray, left by my bed I found a plastic blue clamp which looked liked kids scissors. I secured the bags to my gown. Now I only had the catheter connected to my penis now connected to 3 liters of bright orange piss hanging from my bed. I found that the plastic clip that secured it to my bed made a half decent carry handle. I then tried to reposition the gown as best I could to preserve my modesty or remaining sense of decency as best I could. I slowly edged my feet to the floor realizing this was the first time I had stood vertically since last Wednesday. Left foot, right foot, all good, slowly press off the bed, make sure no tube catches anything, arrh, slight catch on the red blood bag, unhook that, thank god for Mr Morphine and who knows possibly Mr Tramadol lending a hand. I was now standing free from the bed, all I had to do was pick up my external bladder carrying 3 liters of my own piss. I picked it up and steadied myself and suddenly felt a great sense of accomplishment. Take that you bitch Kathy Bates, hours before you had me on the rails, now I was standing and what's more I was mobile, independent and ready to go hunting for calories.

I was lucky that as I exited my C Bay room that Kathy Bates was nowhere to be seen. I asked one of the health assistants where the vending machine was and he pointed me towards the exit from the ward. The first door automatically opened, the second set didn't. A sign said to only press the buzzer once. Could I get away with pressing it once, was someone with a pass going to come along soon. Fuck it I had made it this far, I pressed the buzzer firmly for a full second like someone who was meant to be doing it and expected action.

Suddenly a beep later and the doors were opening. I marched forward out through the doors out of the ward and I was free. Now where was that vending machine, down the end of the walk way. I made my way to the vending machine thinking about what I was going to treat myself to. A refreshing beverage, some soft sweet easily digested source of forbidden calories. I finally made it to find that even though the vending machine was fully stocked that it was out of order and that I should try the vending machines on the other levels. I was not to be denied so I set off. I made it down to floor 4 via the lift only to be denied again but I did come across a security guard that informed me that there was a vending machine on the ground floor that he thought took cash. I had my mission plan and I would not be denied so I set off for the ground floor.

I finally arrived at the ground floor and it was about 1am. I had envisioned being gone for a few minutes but I was not going back empty handed. I finally came across the bank of vending machines that the security guard had referred to and I was almost emotional, these machines contained everything, even a full English breakfast was on offer. My saliva glands kicked into overdrive at the very thought of the possibilities. I started with a full bottle of apple juice. Select the item, confirm coins go in, coins get returned, not valid sale. You must be fucking kidding me, upon examination of the machines I noticed that once again they only took E Payments. I need to find a commercially minded person with E Payment capability. Since I had £20 and wanted less than £8 worth of food, that is a £12 profit for someone, I will not be denied, I was on a mission. As I feverishly walked around the ground floor, I first spied a woman in a tracksuit walking towards me, as I waited for her to be within earshot "Excuse me, I am trying to get some food from theses vending machines, I have £20 I could give you" I caught her eye and immediately she put her hand up and turned and walked the other way. "Not very helpful I thought", the next person was a security guard that didn't seem to hear or see me as I flashed my £20 note as brashly as any stripper from Spearmint Rhino on a slow night, hoping to catch his interest. "Damn, I will not return empty handed" suddenly I saw two moslem woman slowing coming my way. I hid behind one of the columns and tried to make myself look smaller, holding out my £20 note and revealing myself as they came into view of the vending machines for context, I presented my case "I am so sorry to bother you but I am having some trouble getting something to eat and drink from this vending machine, and I only have cash, can you help me, Please?" while they both paused one came forward after a quick word to the other woman who turned out to be her sister. "Yes I can help you, what would you like? " , "Thank You so much for your help. Firstly I would just like a bottle of apple juice". I quickly tried to offer her the £20 note to secure her service but she wouldn't take it. "I have coins as well" I offered and with that we selected the cranberry juice, pressed the button, she presented her phone and then via the magic of robotic automation, a bottle of chilled apple juice dropped down, she retrieved it, handed it to me and with that I quickly forced her to take a few pound coins. My first kill, I was a predator. The next was to get something to eat and the food machine offered everything from a full English breakfast to pasta. I first thought some carbs would be just the thing, **Spaghetti Bolognese 400g A rich bolognese sauce made with minced beef, tomatoes, onions and mushrooms in a tomato and red wine sauce. Served with spaghetti.**

This would be my choice. We selected the item, the machine confirmed our selection and the price of £5.50, please present your card which she did. Nothing happened, what was this? I looked at her and quickly asked "Can we try again?".She confirmed we would, **Spaghetti Bolognese** selected, confirm our selection, present your card and, Nothing again!! I was now becoming desperate and asked if we could try something else as I explained I have been here for 5 days and I have not been able to get anything to eat. So the next selection lets try a **Mini Sausages & Mash 240g** Four tasty pork cocktail sausages in rich beef gravy. Served with buttery mashed potato and peas £3.75. Some nice protein, that would do the trick, I could almost taste the sausages bathed in their divine gravy mixing in the delectable creamy mashed potatoes. I realize that this food was coming out of a vending machine as in retrospect I realize the mashed potatoes probably started out as some sort of powder. I would have been lucky if any of the meat in the sausages hadn't made their way from the remnants of some offal from the floor of some slaughterhouse. At the time it just didn't matter, I was Thor, beast slayer, hunter of calories and I would not be denied. Mini sausages and mash selected, please present card, the whirring of gears and the screen pronounced present card. My compatriot presented her card, more whirring, transaction accepted, more turning of gears then suddenly Nothing!! machine fault, transaction canceled. Nothing!! you must be fucking kidding me, the look of desperation in my face was reflected back at me when my lovely partner in crime responded with "Dont worry I will get you something to eat outside, would you like something from Subway". A miracle I swear had just occurred , God's puerile sense of humor satisfied from viewing my plight over the last few hours from on high had resulted in him offering a tip for my comedy routine in the form of the lovely understanding Angel of a lady offering to get me food. "Please take my £20 as I would love a meatball sandwich, please take it" She said no and to wait there while she and her sister would go outside and get me some food. "We will return we promise" It was just then I noticed that her sister who was pregnant was the more hesitant of the two, but both were angels as far as I was concerned, "Yes I will wait here for you, Thankyou so much". As I found a chair and sat down opposite the vending machine that had denied me, I thought how amazing it was that these two demure moslem woman would be my saviors. Two slight women, the taller one being no more that 5 feet 5 inches tall would be the ones that would help complete my quest. I was thinking that their initial reticence and wide eyed looks on their face when they first saw me was due to the fact that I am 6'4 and hence the height difference until I suddenly saw my own reflection in the glass of the vending machine. "Oh my God what they hell. I stood up not recognising the monster that stood

before me, my bag of pus blood and my

green bag of bile freely swinging, my

medium size gown which had splotches of

blood from the many cannula attempts and

the vein or two the blew out spurting blood

over my gown, the gown I had been wearing

for 4 days, and what is more the tube

connecting my penis to my external bladder

contains 3 litres of my own piss, the motion

of my movement bringing my unkempt

genitals into view from time to time as I had

long since lost feeling in my penis. I was

unshaved and my hair, of which I definitely

have a lot, teased out to be standing on end.

At best I looked like a homeless Bad Santa

who had been sleeping rough and carrying 3

liters of my own piss in a clear bag really just set off the whole ensemble.

The two sisters returned about 10 minutes later apologizing that Subway was closed but they had gone to Tesco and purchased me a meatball sandwich and a fruit cup. After trying my best to arrange myself, this task when you are carrying a bag of your own piss connected to your freely hanging penis is no small order. These women then refused to take my money and both wished me well and that I would recover soon. I imagined my state, the fact that I had probably flashed them both without meaning to and not in a Sexy Full Monty way but in a homeless bad Santa bagman from the street type of way. These women were definitely angels given that the sight of me in the reflection of the vending

machine, I would have run a mile no matter

what note I would be flashing.

Chapter 5

A message from Virgil

After I finally came to my senses Tuesday morning, I was a man that had been savaged by the beast itself. It had sucked me in, lacerated me, weakened me and in the last 24 hours used one of its demons to strip my dignity, make me plead openly to any God, person who would listen for pain relief. I had held on to my friend's hand for dear life as the beast had its talons firmly in me it had tried to pull me further down into the inner depths of the inferno, a point beyond salvation. I may have even cried into the hands of my friend, I couldn't be sure, it was all a blur. as I lay there feeling completely sorry for myself I was interrupted with; "Can I take you Vitals" "Can you fuck, why should I let you?" "After I do, I can give you your pain medication". Now that sounds like a deal, I thought. After the blood pressure, temperature, pulse offering of data I was again reminded of the difficulty of giving me drugs intravenously as the nurse once again used my arm as a pin cushion mumbling. There has got to be one around here somewhere? Yes there has to be I thought, heaps of blood seems to come out every time one of your catheters gets caught on something and ripped out.

As I drifted off to Wonderland with Mr Morphine I was reminded of Dante's journey from the Inferno. Just then Mr Morphine spoke to me as Virgil spoke to Dante.

Oddly enough, my Virgil (Mr Morphine) spoke to me of the Kraken rather than Charon since it was my delirious adventure. He told me in soothing terms of the fact that the Kraken itself was not evil and did not have it in for me, his demonic nurse harpy representatives did not live off my pain and suffering, they didn't savor my every indignity and plot to find ways to trick me into thinking I would be receiving pain relief only to have them deny the precious relief from pain at the last minute due to a slow computer, they didn't, even if it felt like they did, they did not, even if it felt like the Harpies did, the Harpy bitches did not said Virgil.

The Kraken was no more evil than the blue whale is to the plankton it consumes while feeding. The fish that continue to feed upon smaller fish in its gut are not its minions meant to bring pain and misery to small fish families, to wreak havoc on plankton just living their lives, loving each other, watching plankton NETFLIX, just trying to get by. The Kraken is an act of God, like Glactus consuming worlds, it does not have anything against the people of earth, it's just out for a walk and something to eat. Virgil had now given me a frame of reference that I could use, this heinous, hateful, tormenting entity with its demonic harpies living off the lifeblood of my misery were not out to get me. It just felt like it.

Every system in nature can be reduced to a set of basic rules that both tormented and tormentee must abide by. Being a closet geek, I thought of this problem like hacking a incredibly messy, old, nasty, defunct, operating system and when I say hacker, I mean a million years ago 9600 Baud sense of the term, for there was a time when I hacked my Dad's bank (upon revealing said act to my father he had me promptly arrested by a friend of his in the force that turned up on his police motorbike after a 10 min talk about the dangers of what I was doing, never hacked anything after that ever again) I was going to work this system out, I would crack the Kraken that was NHS Post Operative Care, I would regain my dignity, I would regain control of my life.

When I looked at the system the one thing that did occur to me was the need for vitals on a 4 hour basis. Even the life sucking harpies had to conform to this rule that vitals needed to be taken every 4 hours. I had to control their ability to take my vitals. It seemed the more this 4 hour routine was kept, the happier their masters were. So I was supposed to be given Morphine every 4 hours so I would link the two, no Mr Morphine, no vitals. I have a plan and could not wait to try it out.

"I need to get your vitals"

"I need my prescribed pain medication"

"I will get it after I get your vitals"

"No I cannot let you take my vitals until you get me my pain meds"

"why not"

"Because after they wear off I find a comfortable spot and reman still until the next round so that my pain cycle does not kick off again:"

"so can I get your vitals"

"not until you get me my pain meds"

"OK then!"

Amazingly, I had just played poker with the beast and won a hand, she dutifully returned with what made me feel like Robert Johnson at the crossroads, selling my soul to satan, vitals were exchanged for Morphine. Hello Virgil, thank you so much for your advice . The monster doesn't just like the misery and despair of my life. "I told you so," said Virgil. As I drifted along with my consort realizing that this was just the first step. I was pain free for 60 minutes at most, I could not just lie here, it felt like a waste and the look on Virgil's face seemed to indicate he expected more. So I have had my gut decimated, I need to get mobile, I need to walk. Yes I need to walk.

Feeling excited at my new found direction I realized this was not as simple as it sounded. I was connected to two drains from my gut, I had a catheter for a penis and my bladder was a bag hanging from the side of my bed. The intravenous drips were pretty much done anyway so I figured out how to disconnect them. I realized I could unhook my external bladder from the bed and my drains were connected to bags which I could attach to my gown. I now had found pressure stocking and extra large grip socks that would prevent me from slipping. I had my plan so as the hour of pain relief that Mr Morphine allowed me came to a close I had my plan. I would retreat to my motionless, pain free state for the next three hours. I had a plan and a date to dance with the Kraken.

"Can I take your vitals" said the nurse, "Can I have my pain meds", "Can I just first get", "No I need my pain meds before I move, if I move it sets of my pain cycle", "Really", "Yes really", "Ok then"

He shoots, he scores, off she goes and she returns with Mr M, I almost happily gave her full access to take my vitals as 50 ml of Mr Morphine was syringed into my mouth and a yellow and green capsule containing 50 mg of Tramadol. I was given 60 minutes of pain free movement at least with the help of Mr T.

Chapter 6

Counting can be tough or Predator or

Prey

It was now Tuesday afternoon and I
was going to get some walking exercise, I
was getting mobile. I first took both my drain
bags, one of blood and pus and the other of
green shit and tied them to my gown. I then
managed to gather up with an external
bladder which meant that I was carrying
about 3kg of my own piss while still being
connected to the bag. I had no intravenous
encumbrances and my green pressure
stockings and walk socks, I was ready to go.
I slid my legs over the edge of the bed, feet

to the floor and pushed off the bed. I was once again vertical. Now where was I going to go? I quickly worked out that the length of the ward was 45m and that if I did that 22 times that would be 1 kilometer. So out I went with all the confidence that Mr Morphine and Mr Tramadol had given me. As I started to walk I kept track in my mind, one length, two lengths, 3 lengths, 4 lengths, 5 lengths, my stomach is starting to hurt a bit, 6 lengths, I have to remember to tape my penis to my leg as the walking is causing it to bang against my leg and while I can't feel it it feels like I am pissing myself as I walk. God this hurts now where was I 10 lengths or is it 11 lengths or is it 12 lengths, God I hope it is 13 lengths and my stomach full of fish hooks on the wash cycle that is starting to feel like spin. God how many fucking lengths did I walk. Get out of my way as I charged down the ward trying to navigate the general traffic. I should go back to 10 lengths, 11 lengths, 12 lengths, fuck this I am going back to my bed. As I hooked my bag of piss onto my bed and rolled onto my bed, I of course caught one of my drains which will make you get up in the morning with a shock. Shit this hurts, I had been walking for 40 minutes and I had no idea how many lengths I had done but what I needed to do now was to lie down and find a free pain position, for in 15 minutes the pain free cover from Mr Morphine would be lifted. I must find the position and then lie dormant waiting for the next 3 hours to pass before Mr Morphine would once again allow me freedom to move about. Mr T while making life a little more manageable didn't really seem to take the edge off the slicing of my gut pain that seemed to come from excessive movement but healing is a process and it was less than a week after my life saving operation.

As I lay there still waiting for the three hours to pass I took stock of my situation again. Most people here don't really care about my pain or my recovery, the NHS is a monster of an organization run by more administrators than caregivers. What is worse from our consumption of shows like ER, House, Dr Strange most of us are under the impression that Doctors and health practitioners are well paid and live very cool flashy lives. The reality is quite different, the chance of a NHS Doctor being able to purchase the Jaeger-LeCoultre Master Ultra Thin Perpetual watch that Dr Strange wears which retails at around £30,000 is about the same as my Harpy of a nurse becoming self aware, developing empathy and apologizing for putting me through hell, in short fat chance. I realized that I was the person that cared the most about my pain and my recovery and I was now part of this monster's ecosystem. I would have to decide the role I was to play within it. I would have to decide whether I was to be a predator or prey. I would have to work out how to survive within this ecosystem and what's more ratchet my way up the food chain. This Harpy was in reality, some young girl, in a low paying job that wasn't very rewarding, she probably had many people she was angry with. Using a bit of life experience and perspective I could see it was not my misery that she fed off but rather her attitude was her own protection against all the shit going on in her own life. The dog eat dog world of working for Europe's largest employer, one of 1,400,000 other employees and she was a caregiver which meant she was severely outnumbered by the number of professional administrators that guide the NHS monster. Her attitude was not a personal vendetta against me but protection from life in general. Suddenly I saw her for what she was, almost a victim of the system. The ecosystem now came into full view and my recent mauling by the beast had been put in perspective. This was the price I had to pay to learn the rules. I was not going to be prey, I was going to become a predator in this ecosystem. The NHS Kraken neither loves or hates, like blue whales feeding on plankton, they are not the evil destroyers of plankton families and culture, cruelly bringing death and disaster to peaceful plankton communities across the world, they are just whales out feeding.

I have to get myself a game plan, plan your work and work your plan was my mantra. They need to take my vitals every 4 hours. The pain meds give me mobility for an hour and if I find a pain free position, I can wait out 3 hours until they next need vitals. I now had a way to exercise, put together my own routine around the 4 hour NHS regimen. So I began, I would get my pain meds, I would get up, start doing laps up and down the ward but despite having won a few math awards at school and having a fair grip on numbers do you think I could keep track of how many times I had gone up and down the ward. As the pain increased, I was sure I was skipping forward my count due to just wanting it over. I needed something to lock me in so I could reliably count my distance. As I came back to my bed once again thinking I had walked somewhere between 20 and 25 laps of the ward. I came across my collection of coins that I had just put into a paper cup. Then the solution dawned upon me. I put 5 pound coins in my cup and waited for the next round of pain meds. The next round of mobility giving pain meds arrived and I was ready. I had my bodily fluid bags attached to my gown, 2 liters of my own piss in one hand and my cup with my 5 pound coins in the other. I slipped the 5 coins into my hand, placed the cup at the end of the ward and I was off. All I had to do was to go down and back up and every time I got back to the cup I would deposit a coin. Down and back up was 88m so every time I deposited my 5 coins, I had walked 440m. So filling the cup and emptying it 3 times would give me 1320m and 4 times 1760 m or just over a mile. I had my system, I had control, I was not a victim, and I was going to recover.

I then felt I needed to find out my weight. I knew that I was 122 kg when I came into the hospital, so I just needed to find out what I weighed now. I needed to find a scale. Of all the gadgets the NHS has on the wards there are no simple scales, there is however a chair you can sit in. You sit in the chair and of course the read out is behind you. I am sure it also cost more than most people's sofas but I learnt that I could kneel on the seat and look backwards at the readout to find my weight. At least the scale seemed accurate. It knew I had arrived last Wednesday and my weight was 122 kg and it was now 118 kg. I had lost 4 kg and to be honest that was 4 kg I definitely did not need. I was thinking that 112 kg would put me back where I was when I was 50, and that meant all my clothes would fit, not a bad thing. Maybe a bit ambitious but one needs a goal. Now I needed a goal of distance to get my arse out of bed, use the freedom the pain meds gave me to get mobile and start my recovery.

A Marathon, what else, I could calculate how many meters. My 5 coins and a cup method would make sure I didn't happen to short count my trips back and forward as I did find a certain amount of pain would make the brain come up with phantom trips in order to get the whole process over quicker. Now as it turned out, walking up and down the ward several times a day, 12 times to cover one kilometre was proving a little disruptive so I ventured out of the ward to find the length of the walkway outside the ward that was exactly 120m so that would be 220m down and back. Now if I emptied and filled my cup with 5 coins twice I would be doing 2.2km a time. It was taking me about 15 min to drop 5 coins so this would keep me out for 30 minutes given my deep breathing exercises that were also a pain. This would give me enough time to get back into bed to find my pain free position and then remain still for 3 hours until my next round of pain meds. This was my plan and I would not deviate from this plan, no matter how nice the nurse might be about wanting my vitals, no pain meds, no vitals, this is how I tamed the beast and became a predator for my recovery.

No one is going to care more about your recovery than you and you know your own life better than anyone else. You should be at least as well informed about what is going on with you as anyone else, it's your recovery for christ sake, you have to take ownership and tame the beast. You are a part of the ecosystem during recovery and the role you wish to play is your choice. I am a predator hunting my recovery and that is what drove me.

I unfortunately was still wearing the same gown from last Friday, still had not had a shave, still had not had my bed sheets changed and still with all my tubes looked like Bad homeless Santa with a predilection for exposing myself. I had to do something about my cave because my cave was a mess. I requested to have a shower and her response was "Oh all right then" which I thought was strange since I was thinking that out of self interest she would want me too as I was starting to become aware of my own scent which is never a good thing.

The nurse gave me a plastic bag with shampoo, 3 razors which I thought was odd, soap, two towels and two large gowns as per my request. As I closed the door to the shower space and took off my gown and it was only then that I truly appreciated how far I had let this go, the blood stains, the green stain, the brown stain which I thought odd since I had not been able to pass anything since I arrived. Contrary to what my Doctors professed, I didn't believe my body could turn apple juice and strawberry yogurt into decent stools. When I took the gown off it could almost stand by itself, crusty would be the word I would use. There was no wash cycle on earth that was going to make that wearable again so in the bin it went. I got under the water for the first time since I had arrived almost a week beforehand and felt reborn as I soaped myself, not wanting to look down as I washed one week's worth of myself away. A cleansing experience in so many ways. I lathered myself three times in all and washed my face feeling my long whiskers which were long enough to become soft to the touch. I now dried myself off, put my two gowns on, one for the front and one for the back, no more flashing my genitals to all and sundry, I attached my bags of blood and green bile, grabbed my bag of my own piss and made my way to the toilet for a well deserved shave.

I had never really appreciated companies like Harry's and Gillete and all the work they put into the modern razor. I had been given three disposable razors and some shaving cream. I was looking forward to a freshly shaved face. I lathered my face, first razor, a couple of strokes and the razor was filled with my whiskers although none seemed to be removed from my face, in fact all I seemed to have done is to mush the shaving cream into what I could best describe as homeless Santa's beard. Second razor, same result, third razor same result, I had managed to go through three razors without seemingly having removed any whiskers from my face. To the suppliers of razors to the NHS, "Fuck You". I really mean it as the razors did seem to contain a blade of sorts. To make something that looks like a disposable razor, had a handle like a disposable razor but possessed no ability to remove whiskers at all and then managing to sell them to the NHS is a true coup. The fact that the nurse had given me a bag with three razors now seemed to make sense. Unfortunately, it could have been a big bag of razors and it would not have made any difference. The last thing to do now I felt was to clean my ears as they felt a little gunky. I don't know why being in hospital seems to increase the rate of ear wax production substantially but I could feel that my ears needed a cleaning. I managed to get some wet wipes and some of those wooden sticks you stir coffee with so I could clean my ears. The first insertion of the stick pulled out an amount of bright orange wax that even surprised me. I grabbed a new wet wipe, wrapped it around the stick and proceeded into the other ear and oh my god what came out was more like a small colony with orange being mixed in with grey and black. Had some insect laid something in my ear? I grabbed another wet wipe and went into the first ear again and it was like I never even went in the first time with a huge covering or orange wax covering the wipe, I wondered how in the hell this had happened. I then dug back into the other ear again and fortunately it returned just orange wax and not bug larvae which was a relief. In all I went into both ears 5 times before I managed to pull out a wet wipe not covered in earwax. You may be wondering why I bring this up, well if you have spent any times on the recovery wards you well hear this scenario often

Nurse "Good morning Peter how are you feeling this morning"

Patient "Hello, no I am not aware of anyone stealing things from me"

Nurse "No I asked how are you feeling today"

Patient "We I am healing just fine but my anus is still bothering me"

Nurse "Well I am not here to look at your anus right now but to get your blood pressure"

Patient "You want to see my old treasures, I haven't heard them called that before but if you must"

Nurse "I just want your blood pressure Peter"

Patient "Oh I think you are a treasure too but what do you want from me?"

It becomes clear very quickly that given the number of elderly patients of which I suppose I am one (Over 50) it is not that they are all deaf or hard of hearing, it's just that their ears are full of wax. I fortunately was able to remove the ear wax that the ear wax fairies had dumped in my ears while on the ward but most of the patients are packing enough to lubricate a small truck. For all the money wasted on razors you would think one nurse tasked with cleaning the ears of the patients on the wards would prove a major boost to better communication between patients and staff on the wards. Better communication, less stress, less stress better for everyone concerned. Just an observation as I had noticed many patients seem to complain of partial deafness when on the ward. I think the outbreak of ward deafness might be miraculously cured by one nurse with a decent supply of cotton buds. It would be a great job as she would have the power to give the deaf people back their hearing. A nurse and a few cotton buds and miracles of hearing could follow, just a thought.

In any event I had my first shower, I had control of my bags of bodily fluids, I would hunt for a real razor later. I was starting to take hold of my situation and decided I would be a predator in this ecosystem, and I also made friends with one of the Healthcare assistants Salome, she even changed my bedsheets, my cave was now clean and so was I. I wouldn't just survive, I would prosper.

Chapter 7

The making of my marathon and the

price of exit

One of the conditions of leaving the NHS Post Operative care is the natural passing of stool. Now in all my years of being a carnivore I was always under the assumption that to produce stool one needed to eat and by eat I mean real food like bread, meat, cheese all those things I believe now to be carcinogenic. I always thought by this logic that stools from these foods then must be carcinogenic as well. I never really considered the consumption of 100 ml of yogurt or chicken broth to be the stuff of good stools but the doctors looking after me seemed to believe that consumption of this "food" would produce stool. Given my difficulty in producing stool on a diet of yogurt and broth they had decided enemas were the way ahead. After a solid rectal exam the morning before to announce that nothing was there but the x-ray showed some stool, the next morning the nurse showed up ready to administer my enema. The nurse was new, Filipino, full makeup, bright red lipstick and a big smile. She came to the end of my bed and announced, I will be giving you your enema in about 5 minutes. "Thank you I said, I am looking forward to it". A few minutes later she returned to say that she has to do something but will be back soon to give me an enema "Thankyou" again I said. I went for a quick 1 km walk as I thought a shot of gravity, God's natural enema assistant could not hurt. Once I returned from my walk she was there. "I am ready to give you your enema now, " she said. "Wonderful I said"

As she drew the privacy curtain around she once again loudly announced "I am here to give you an enema, you should lie down on the bed and relax and I will administer the enema by pumping the fluid into your anus"

"You know I said, I think everybody in the room including myself is well aware of what is just about to happen without you having to explain it in detail. ok she said with a smile. As I lay on the bed, " please bring your knees to your chest as I am going to insert the end of the bottle" "I really think they don't need to hear exactly what you are doing".

"Sorry" she said with a smile which I thought was interesting as this woman who was holding a bottle of fluid connected to a tube she was inserting into my anus could still muster a big smile and look my right in the eye while she was doing it. It was like she loved her job. As she pushed am pumped away I could feel all sort of indescribable uncomfortable feelings as I had spent my life as a thumb out kind of guy, not that I am homophobic or anything, I have experienced the request from girlfriends in the past but I can honestly say whatever was done the last thing I ever felt was, can't wait to do that again no matter how hot she was or how much she seemed to enjoy doing it to me.

"All done" she announced with a big smile,

"Just lay there for a few minutes and relax" I couldn't fault her bedside manner, I thought. As the fluid made its way like a wave machine around my bowels I felt that sense of foreboding nausea that seemed to make sense to me at any rate. After laying there for 10 min and tentatively making sure that shifting to the vertical would not result in a stream of shit down my leg, I decide to take myself to the bathroom. Given that at this stage I was 33 km into my Marathon I had probably given gravity a good chance to work its magic on my stools. As I turned out of my Bay A room, wouldn't you know the mens bathroom is in the middle of being cleaned. Never before have I witnessed this but with 300ml of fluid washing around my bowel the cleaner decided to clean the male toilet. Now this is one of those times where depending on your mental state you may believe that the NHS monster and its minions are out to get you but even though it seems like a conspiracy to have me shit myself midmorning in full view of everyone on the ward, you can't jump to conclusions. So as I started to prance around like I was doing the latest Tik Tok dance I reasoned to myself. The world does not hate me, I have just come across the remaining 80% of the population just trying to get by. The man cleaning the men's bathroom is not out to get me by timing his cleaning schedule to coincide with the exact time I need to use the bathroom, I am sure cleaning the toilets at this time was not part of a plan to screw me over but his job. A job that I observed him doing fairly well. Did the nurse who administered my enema have it in for me by timing the enema just at the right time to coincide with the toilet cleaning schedule and her smile and pleasant demeanour wasn't a sarcastic front for her true self drawing pleasure from the idea that I would shit myself mid-morning in the middle of the ward in front of everyone just because my body doesn't turn yogurt and chicken broth into real shit. These people were just trying to get by, doing their jobs with a positive attitude with probably more enthusiasm that I could muster. It just felt like it at that moment. "Bathroom is ready" "Thank God, as I sat down on a freshly cleaned toilet seat in a the freshly cleaned toilet as I emptied the shitty soup the had been washing around my bowels for the last 10 minutes I thought to myself, I should thank the man who cleaned this toilet, really I should for I have not felt so clean inside and out in years in my nice freshly cleaned toilet. Thankyou Mr Cleaning man, thank you and thank you to the cheerful Nurse Raissa who made getting an enema as pleasant as I imagine it could be.

As I ventured out of the toilet to return to my bed I passed the nurse and she asked if I was ok and I told her that I had just got rid of the 300 ml of fluid that she had recently put up my anus. "You didn't open your bowels properly" she said "Maybe another enema". "No, it's ok." I started to explain the whole yogurt, broth equals stools concept when she immediately said "I will tell the doctor straight away, maybe you will need another enema, because the enema has medicine that opens your bowls you will see another one will definitely work". Once again, this Nurse Raissa was one of the angels just trying to help. I imagined she put on full makeup every day she went to work. She is a nurse because she likes to help people, sometimes she gets to help people by giving them medicine and this makes her happy. Enema has medicine in it to help me open my bowels which is healthy. This is one of the 80% and definitely part of 50% of the 80% that tries to make the world a better place as much as she can. During this whole episode an interesting notion did occur to me, when the doctor said that when consuming small quantities of yogurt and chicken broth that he expected a certain amount of stool to be produced. Maybe most people can make shit out of basically nothing. Vegans for example must be able to crank out huge amounts of stool on nothing more than celery and water. New age diets not containing meat at all allow certain types of people to produce glorious stools on nothing more than some lettuce leaves and a pot of Greek yogurt.   There is also the possibility that some people are able to make shit out of nothing and some people only make shit out of real food. One for the social scientists and the nutritionists to consider. I completed my marathon the following day and glory be after weighing myself before and after an enema, I managed to get rid of approximated 200g of stool by my weight calculations. Not really the movement I was after but progress, nonetheless.

What is a cannula?

A cannula is a fine tube inserted into a vein, usually in the back of your hand or arm, using a small fine needle. The needle is removed, and the tube is left inside your vein. The cannula has 1 or more connectors which allow staff to give fluids and medication (drugs) directly into your bloodstream. Sometimes a cannula may be inserted into your foot, leg or other part of your body. A cannula is sometimes called a Venflon.

What care should be taken when my cannula is inserted?

To reduce the risk of infection the nurse or doctor who will insert your cannula should clean their hands and wear gloves and an apron. The skin around the area will be cleaned. All cannulas are used only once and come from the manufacturer sterilized and in a sealed packet. The packaging is opened just before use. A note will be made in your healthcare record of the date and time when your cannula was inserted.

During my time inside the beast I had maybe 20 cannulas inserted into my arms. What they don't say is that the art of inserting a cannula is actually a medical skill. It's very much like when a doctor picks up an ophthalmoscope or one of those things with the bright blinding lights, pokes it towards your eye and then says "keep your eye still and don't look at me". A trained medical professional is able to look around the back of your eyeball and can tell you all sorts of things, such as the health of your optic nerve, even if you are a diabetic. A regular person won't be able to see shit, I know I have tried, it's a real skill to be able to use one of these things. Putting in a cannula like using an ophthalmoscope is a real skill that obviously the book says every nurse and doctor should know how to do but this is just not the case. As it turns out I have particularly difficult veins to cannulate so during my time given my need for intravenous antibiotics I need working cannulas. This turned my arms into pin cushions for all and sundry, what I did learn is that I would be a crap heroin addict always slowing the party down. Has Wayne spiked his vein yet? Nearly, almost there. "You said that 5 minutes ago" lets try the other arm."isnt heroin great" "Yeah real great almost there" "Damn missed the vein, you guys go ahead and I will catch up, got to be a vein around here somewhere, they made it look so fucking easy in the movie trainspotting". With all the attempts to cannulate me one really stood out. It was on day 17 of my stay and I had 3 cannulas in the last 2 days to try and provide me with intravenous antibiotics and I was accordingly unimpressed. A doctor came to my bedside and announced he was there to cannulate me and feeling a little bit down given my gut was feeling a bit sore I grunted acknowledgement. He proceeded to use the ultrasound without any cooperation from myself as I had been trying my best to assist his predecessors but at that moment I had had enough of being pricked. In a moment it was in and he was securing it with the associated bandages, (notably without any of the children's bears that seem to come with the bandage) this man meant business and within 30 seconds he had the cannula in, flushed and working, I complimented him and he replied "It's not hard, just needed to be done properly" and boy it was done properly. I asked him his name and he replied Doctor Tom, "Where are you from?" done. He reminded me that a true medical professional comes with skills and abilities us non medical types do not possess. Within all professions, you have differing levels of skills and abilities and while previously I had medical staff from the 2nd and 3rd division, I had just witnessed skills from a premier league professional and it really stood out. I just want to say hi to Doctor Tom from Sheffield Medical school who definitely knew what he was doing and should be regarded with pride by the NHS. They do in fact do things better up north. His cannula lasted until the end of my time there. If only I had Dr Tom do my cannula when I first arrived, my Green Button experience would have been turbo charged. Go Sheffield Medical and top marks to Dr Tom.

Chapter 8

Heaven versus Hell and where to get your haircut

During my stay I got the opportunity to be housed in both the David Evans Ward and the St Mary Abbot Ward or SMA as it is known. I must admit the amateur cosmologist inside me was fascinated by the experience. I believe I got to see the very birth of two small proto-societies, one destined to be hell and the other destined to be heaven. My experience in life has left me with the following observational truth, that 10% of people are amazing, inspiring, benevolent, giving, empathetic beings capable of acts that keep us moving forward as a species, provide us with acts that touch our hearts during those songs that all make us hold our breath. It is like the acts of James Garner in the Notebook at the end of the movie, acts that show the best of us, of what we are capable of. Then there is the bottom 10% of us, selfish, malevolent, self-obsessed, nasty pieces of shit that cause 90% if not 100% of all the problems that infect our society. Then there is the rest of us, 80% who are just trying to get by, do a bit of living, do not rock the boat too much, enjoy a few simple pleasures that we are more than happy to pay for before we shuffle off this mortal coil. If you want to break it down further there is a gradient between the upper 10% and the bottom 10% that influences those closest to these extremities. In my experience this is how society is made up and I have collected a set of rules for social development. People within a society are called to act using after being prodded some way into action by a situation. It is the way in which people respond to these calls to action that dictate how a society develops.

Top 10%	**Angels**		
	Benevolent	Inspiring	Giving
The Rest of Society	Good, decent people		
	Most of society sits somewhere here		
	Evil bastards		
Bottom 10%	**Demons**		
	Selfish	Malevolent	Self Obsessed

Societal Environmental Decisions by Angels

or Arseholes Conditions

SEDAA Conditions

1. Will I have to pay a penalty if I

   don't act

2. Will this action benefit me

3. Is the action covered by a rule or

   regulation so I can say I did my

   job

   while taking no action

4. Does this action make common sense

   5. Does someone else need

   my help

It is the order in which these laws are

interpreted by the individual that results in

the way a society develops. The only thing

that really matters is the way in which the individual ranks the first two conditions when approaching a call to action.

Scenario

For example, we have a situation where there is a person who is in a stupid amount of pain, a person whose history you are familiar with who is pleading with you for pain relief. The person's distress is negatively affecting the well-being of others around them, and you have the pain killer in your hand and are able to provide relief.

Bottom 10% analysis.

1. Who will the action benefit me

   NO

2. Is the action covered by a rule or regulation that I can hide behind

   YES

This response to actions over time results in a hell type environment developing.

Top 10% analysis.

1. Does someone else need my help

    Yes

2. Does this action make common sense

    Yes

This response arc to the scenario will result in the development of a heaven type environment development.

This is what I found to be the difference between the David Evans Ward and the SMA. The problem is that it only takes a few demons mixed in with a few angels to still create a hell type environment. One of the things that really struck me on the SMA were the angelic Nurses and Healthcare assistants that really made the SMA bearable. While the demons tried their very best to make life unbearable for all those around them including their work colleagues at times, the angels made the place bearable against the chaos created by the lesser beings. The angels that I recall are the lovely Healthcare Assistant Salome, then Nurse Joyce that made the last two weeks of my stay bearable. I must also mention Nurse Raissa who enthusiastically gave me quite a few enemas whose technique made them bearable, I thank you. There was also Kamil who found me XL socks when no one else could and Nurse Shauna and the Senior Nurse who ran the David Evans Ward who made my stay there so enjoyable. It was a pleasure to see how a different attitude could change the entire atmosphere of a place of work. You are a true credit to the NHS.

The other thing that seemed really obvious to me was there seemed to be a lot of miscommunications between hospital staff and patients and not forgetting the ear wax pixy problem, some large A4 pads with some markers might be helpful. Just because someone is old, and even if they are hard of hearing, doesn't mean they cannot read. Subtitles have been a big hit over the years and have allowed movies in many languages to be enjoyed by many. Here is my idea, A4 pads, real time subtitles for real time communication between nursing staff and patients. Once again just

take it out of the razor budget and you would
definitely improve communications and
hence lower anxiety between patients and
staff.

Once I came to terms with the fact that
I was part of the NHS Kraken ecosystem I
learnt that the wards are 44m long, the
walkways are 120m long and if you take a
wide berth and do circuits of the ground floor
walkways, if you do 5 laps you have walked
1.25 km. I also found out that Chelsea and
Westminster has a disused radio station
pod, it has a movie theatre on the third floor
and unfortunately, try as I might, I never got
to see a movie there. During my exploration
of the skeleton of the beast I discovered in
the back on the second floor, a room you
might mistake for storage, the Alto Hair

Salon run by a fascinating lady from Clapham of Italian heritage called Emma that has been cutting hair of many of the patients, doctors and administrators of the beast itself for years. She has many fascinating stories that she passed on to me while I had my hair cut by her. Some of the accommodations that she has made for some of the patients that exist on the more ethereal plains of consciousness are truly astounding. The beast takes all and sundry in and Emma gets to cut their hair. If you are staying in the C & W and are in need of a haircut, I thoroughly recommend her.

I urge anyone that is in the clutches of NHS post operative care that you get to decide the role you will play in the ecosystem you find yourself in. The beast will feed no matter what you do so your choice is to be prey or predator. You can allow all the variables of the human condition to rule over your recovery or you can take charge, show interest in the beast and carve out your own recovery.

I must say that while some of the nurses I came across during my time definitely used logical thought and compassion as a fall back to more petty, opportunistic methods of dealing with patient care. There were others that made all the difference and were part of the team that allowed the beast to save my life and allow me to recover. It may seem incredible but the staff of the NHS that I saw who would use common sense to direct their actions would find themselves butting up against poorly thought through mantra created by those who don't know and executed by those who don't care. The NHS currently employs nearly 1.4 million full time equivalent people making it the largest employer in England and the largest employer in Europe. At the moment 1 in 17 workers in England work for the NHS. They predict by 2035 that it will rise to 1 in 11. It is the equivalent of a giant beast neither loving or hating, acting with love or malevolence, just the act of it feeding is an act of God, like the blue whale when it feeds it can be seen to be a savior or a destroyer depending on where you sit on the food chain. These perceived acts of God, creates micro communities and possibly micro religions as plankton may see blue whales as inherently evil destroyers of worlds. It is your job when you get sucked into the ecosystem that is the NHS is to decide how you are going to navigate its ecosystem, whether you will be a victim or a predator. Whether you will fall victim to its nastier minions (demons) or learn to navigate around them and to avail yourself of its more benevolent representatives (angels). It's heaven and hell all mixed together but one thing is for sure, you get to choose your place in its ecosystem. It renders healthcare to millions each year and one hopes it saves considerably more lives than it kills but it is not going away anytime soon.

To the Kraken, you were a worthy opponent and an awesome hack and in reality, you saved my life after I paid it a visit late one

Wednesday night and for that I owe the big

monster thanks.

Chapter 9

Your Recovery and Survival is up to You

If you are not the most interested person in your recovery you need not worry because you are already dead and have made it to heaven where your God has placed an Angel in charge of your healthcare. Back on earth things are a little different. You must be the person most interested in your recovery and by that, I mean you must become aware of which medications you have been prescribed and why and how much of each medication you are to take and how often. To think that those looking after you are incapable of making a mistake is naïve. One thing I found to be very helpful was putting together my own table. I had a list of the painkillers, oral morphine 5ml and Tramadol 50mg every 4 hours. I would suggest linking up giving your vitals with the taking of your medication every 4 hours, given you are probably going to be woken up whether you like it or not. The following table is an example of what I kept for myself.

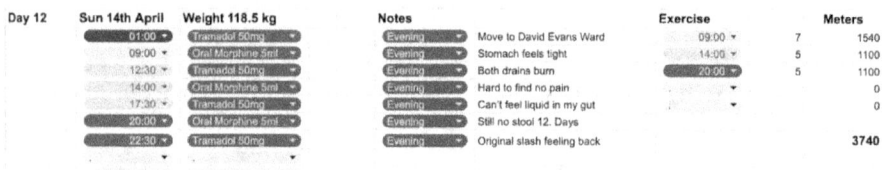

Day 12	Sun 14th April	Weight 118.5 kg		Notes			Exercise			Meters
	01:00	Tramadol 50mg		Evening		Move to David Evans Ward	09:00		7	1540
	09:00	Oral Morphine 5ml		Evening		Stomach feels tight	14:00		5	1100
	12:30	Tramadol 50mg		Evening		Both drains burn	20:00		5	1100
	14:00	Oral Morphine 5ml		Evening		Hard to find no pain				0
	17:30	Tramadol 50mg		Evening		Can't feel liquid in my gut				0
	20:00	Oral Morphine 5ml		Evening		Still no stool 12. Days				
	22:30	Tramadol 50mg		Evening		Original slash feeling back				3740

You must make sure you keep notes of the time for everything that happens to you. You should ask questions if you do not understand something, you should be able to recognise what your medication looks like. They are all different colors and have different markings on them so that they can be identified.

You can easily download an app on your phone that will help you identify what you are being given. You should always remember that the NHS is staffed by Demons as well as Angels and as caring and attentive as the Angels are, the uncaring, flippant, power hungry, inconsiderate and often incompetent Demons are always lurking. That is why you must always be the most interested person in your recovery. If you care to have a look at some of the pictures I took during my time in hospital, please go to Instagram and look for "5 Coins and a Cup".

https://www.instagram.com/5coinsandacup/. Some of the pictures are fairly graphic so you have been warned.

One must remember that due to the size of the NHS beast it consumes patients and discharges without feeling or interest due to the fact that it is just a process, a giant of a process that saves the lives of many more people than it kills, and like all giant ecosystems you have to decide what role you are going to play once you are part of it. If you are a patient here are some notes that you might find helpful.

- **When it comes to gowns wear two, put the first one on and then wear the second one like a coat, preserves your dignity and prevent accidental exposure**
- **Make sure when you wear the pressure stockings but remember they are slippery so always wear the grip socks with them.**

- None of the vending machines accept cash including the Costa Coffee on the ground floor so make sure you have your phone app or contact debit card handy
- The only person who does accept cash is the concession man who makes his way on to the wards every day. He not only can get you anything you need if you ask him and he takes cash.
- The lovely Emma who can give you a haircut is located on the second floor but if you ask the concession man he can organize an appointment for you. Her number is 0203 315 8681.
- The walkways are 120 m long, the wards are 44 m long but I would suggest walking exercise be conducted on the walkways. It is also worth noting that 4 times around the ground floor loop is 1 km.

About the Author

Wayne Harburn survived a gastric perforation with chemical peritonitis one evening after consuming some warm ham and cheese rolls. The NHS saved him, but his life experience and logical approach allowed him not only to survive the NHS postoperative monster but thrive. He left 5kg lighter with better exercise habits. He completed a walking marathon and half a step marathon while he was there. His blood pressure was last measured at 130/90 and he intends to remember the lessons he learnt and hopefully not revisit the NHS recovery monster again anytime soon. He is also grateful to all the people who saved his life that fateful Thursday when he wandered into the A & E and those angels who helped so much in his recovery. To the demons, well, you are still in hell and he escaped...

www.ingramcontent.com/pod-product-compliance
Lightning Source LLC
Chambersburg PA
CBHW051311220526
45468CB00004B/1299